CBD HEMP OIL

AND

ARTHRITIS

THE ULTIMATE GUIDE TO MARIJUANA AND ARTHRITIS

DAVID QUINTIN MD

DISCLAIMER

Please note that every attempt has been made to provide accurate, up to date and reliable information. No warranties of any kind are expressed or implied. Readers acknowledge that the author or publisher is not liable for any usage of the content of this book. Ensure to consult your doctor or any proven licensed physician before practicing.

TABLE OF CONTENT

CHAPTER 1

WHAT IS ARTHRITIS

Arthritis comes from the Greek word arthro means "joint" plus -itis or "inflammation". Thus, it is a health condition relating to inflammation or swelling of the joints.

Although any part of the body can be inflamed with arthritis, usual areas that it weakens are the back, neck, hip, knee, or feet. Some conditions can be devastating and even bring life-threatening complications as it may affect other parts of the body like the muscles, bones and internal organs.

CHAPTER 2

OVERVIEW OF ARTHRITIS

When most people think about arthritis, they largely associate it with the elderly. There is some factual basis to this assumption, as the disease is by far most common among senior citizens. However, it can actually affect people of all ages, including very young children. It is also common for people to think of arthritis as a single disease, but it actually encompasses more than 100 different diseases, many of which are quite different.

While there are over a hundred types of arthritis and some of them affect the body in vary different ways, there are also a number of symptoms that are common across the different kinds of arthritis. The disease typically affects the various joints in the body, commonly causing inflammation, swelling, and general stiffness in the affected joints. Among senior citizens, osteoarthritis is the most common type of arthritis, often affecting the knees.

In addition to symptoms that affect mobility and the joints, causing general movement issues, there are also a number of other symptoms. This includes fever, extreme tiredness, hunger, weight loss, dry eyes, and Crepitus.

Crepitus, is a condition where simple movements result in a crackling or popping sound coming from the joints. This is one reason that people often associated cracking ones fingers with arthritis, as they do share similarities, although in the case of cracking fingers, it is not a direct cause of arthritis.

It is most common for arthritis to affect joints, but certain types of arthritis can also affect the joints and cause skin issues, like rashes or scaly lesions on the body. It is also often related to chronic pain, with people experiencing pain in a number of parts of their body.

The most commonly used definition for arthritis is an inflammation of the joints. The joints of the body are where two bones connect allowing the limbs to bend for movement purposes. Arthritis causes the joints to swell which makes the bones stiff and lessens the flexibility of your movement. It is important to note that arthritis is not a single disease.

There are well over 100 rheumatic diseases that cause pain, swelling and stiffness in the joints that arthritis describes. To make it plain there are many different types of arthritis and many different causes for arthritis.

For example osteoarthritis (degeneration of the joints disease)is a form of arthritis and the most common cause of arthritis is hereditary, if a parent suffered from this disease chances are it will get passed on to the children.

CHAPTER 3

CAUSES OF ARTHRITIS

Arthritis is an intensely agonizing condition that has effects on many of us all around the world. It causes joint redness, which in several cases is a source of agony that is virtually insufferable.

There are lots of risk factors that puts one at the mercy of arthritis. Though doctors have known about these dangers for many years, many patients are not conscious of them.

By becoming conscious of the risks of arthritis, you can take the required cares to avoid being forced to suffer because of this unpleasant condition.

Medical professionals have identified four main risk factors of arthritis which they have reckoned to be non-modifiable. This implies that it is not possible to modify them. The four factors that can't be modified are gender, age, ethnicity, and genetics.

Gender: this is one of the commonest, but astonishing risk factors of arthritis. It's a famous fact that more women than men are influenced by arthritis. In addition, ladies are likely to notice the effects of a selection of forms of arthritis. Though men are not fully immune, arthritis is way more ordinarily seen in women.

Age: this is an arthritis risk factor that comes as barely a surprise to the general public. The chance of developing arthritis increases with age. This is particularly true for osteoarthritis. Customarily arthritis risk increases seriously after the age of forty

Ethnicity: is another non-modifiable risk factor of arthritis. Though this factor is comparatively minor, professionals have still seen some correlations between ethnicity and the development of arthritis. The fourth factor is genetics. Certain inherited genes have been shown to extend arthritis risk. More research must be finished to establish how ethnicity and genetics are related to arthritis.

There are some factors of arthritis that can't be modified, without regard for what you do. However, there are more factors that you can change to ward off the development of arthritis.

Obesity: One such factor is obesity. Excess weight can increase the danger of developing arthritis in the knees, hips, and hands. Weight is particularly a risk factor for ladies. Even a mere ten pounds can raise your possibility of developing arthritis.

Others: Two other non-modifiable factors are joint damage and infection. Any sort of injury or infection that has effects on the joints has the capability to trigger redness. Occupation also becomes a risk factor, because work-related stress can frequently lead to arthritis.

Knowing the chance factors of arthritis will make sure that you are thinking about methods to stop the commencement of this condition before it essentially occurs. Though certain non-modifiable risk factors can't be modified, other factors can be modified to put the chances of being touched by arthritis in your favor.

CHAPTER 4: TYPES OF ARTHRITIS

The knowledge of arthritis especially its symptoms will greatly give you the edge on how to handle the situation. The types of arthritis are so numerous to explain in just one book. I however have done my best to explain the most commonly known types.

Osteoarthritis

Osteoarthritis develops from the wearing away of joint cartilage. It is degenerative in nature and the substantial damage caused by excessive strain on the joints and its bordering tissues is characterized by:

• pain

• soreness

• swelling

• difficulty of movement

In its early stages, osteoarthritis is rarely symptomatic and mostly non-inflammatory. It develops slowly and is difficult to detect because it affects only a minimum number of joints. More often than not, osteoarthritis strikes the:

- hands

- hips

- knees

- spine

Advancing age increases the risk of acquiring osteoarthritis. Trauma to the joints, obesity and repetitive joint use comprise the other risk factors of the disease.

Rheumatoid arthritis

Rheumatoid arthritis is a type of inflammatory disease. Generally, it causes intense pain and loss of motion in the particular joint it chooses to attack.

In rheumatoid arthritis, the immune system plays a big part in the development of the disease. When a certain type of reaction triggers a rheumatoid arthritis attack, the result would be unbearable pain in and around the joints.

Rheumatoid arthritis occurs when the synovium, the cell lining within the joint, is mistakenly damaged by the bodys' own immune system.

This type of arthritis is a chronic autoimmune syndrome which is potentially disabling. It is often marked by:

• joint pain

• joint incapacity

• swelling

• stiffness

Rheumatoid arthritis manifests itself over a period of a few months. However, for some, the disease appears overnight. Accelerated onset of rheumatoid arthritis does not mean the individual is at greater risk of the progression of the disease. Rheumatoid arthritis can lasts for years without symptoms. But rheumatoid arthritis is an illness that progresses and has the potential to cause joint destrution and functional disability.

Rheumatoid arthritis is difficult to pin down at its onset due to the minimal number of symptoms. The causes of this type of arthritis are still unknown, but physicians are pointing to heredity as one of its chief causes.

Rheumatoid arthritis is very common in people aged 20 to 45 years of age, although this disease could occur to a person regardless of his age.

People who are suffering from rheumatoid arthritis can't do what a normal person does in terms of physical endeavors such as walking, running, swimming, and exercising. And because of this, the family and friends of the patients with rheumatoid arthritis becomes affected as well.

Rheumatoid arthritis can be caused by a number of factors. While it is rather hard even for the doctors to tell their patient what actually makes them contract the disease, the most common of all factors are listed below:

Viruses, Fungi, and Bacteria have long been suspected to be the root causes of rheumatoid arthritis. But then again, it hasn't been proven that they alone are sufficient to cause the disease. What is certain is that viruses, fungi, and bacteria play a certain role in the development of the disease, as they trigger the body's immune system to act. Therefore, it cannot be ruled out that these infectious agents may have something to do with rheumatoid arthritis.

There are also studies showing that rheumatoid arthritis can be inherited. There have been worldwide researches performed to seek the main cause of this disease. And with that many researches conducted, all of experts behind them can't rule genetics as a factor.

In a certain group of patients who suffers from rheumatoid arthritis, it was found out that a number of them have family members who are suffering from the disease in one way or another. This had caused scientists to assume that certain types of rheumatoid arthritis can be transferred genetically.

Because rheumatoid arthritis involves the immune system, it is reasonable to assume that certain allergens cause the antibodies to attack the joints. Allergens fall under the environmental factors that could trigger the disease. These could be the food you eat, exposure to certain types of bacteria in the air, and the deficiency of certain types of vitamins in the body.

It is therefore important that a series of consultations with a health expert is carried out so that it becomes easy for them to determine what triggers a particular rheumatoid arthritis attack. Defining one's allergen is very helpful in preventing the disease.

One other cause of rheumatoid arthritis would be the changes in one's hormones. For the females, it was found out that during pregnancy, their levels of progesterone and estrogen becomes relatively high. However, after giving birth, it drastically decreases. This is one of the reasons why rheumatoid arthritis often happens in a woman after child birth.

On the flip side, some mothers have experienced improved rheumatoid arthritis condition during the entire length of their pregnancy. But after the time the baby is born, they experience a certain degree of flare up.

There have been relevant studies that show smoking tobacco can increase a person's risk of developing rheumatoid arthritis, now or at any time in the future.

On the other hand, for those people who already have rheumatoid arthritis and still continue to smoke, their chances of having an attack are higher than those who don't. There are certain substances found inside a tobacco that triggers the attack.

The difficulty in diagnosing rheumatoid arthritis in its early stages would be the fact that there is not a single test for this type of disease.

The fact that its symptom may also differ from one patient to another is one more reason why it becomes hard for doctors to assume that the disease a patient suffers from is in fact, rheumatoid arthritis. The mere diagnosis of this disease requires a series of tests in the form or x-rays, blood tests, CRP, and SED rate.

Juvenile arthritis

Children can also be afflicted by a type of arthritis known as juvenile arthritis. It is the most common form of arthritis that besets children. The three major kinds of juvenile arthritis are:

- pauciarticular (affecting only a minimum number of joints)
- polyarticular (involving more than several joints)
- systematic (impacting the whole body)

Indicators of juvenile rheumatoid arthritis are different for each child, and a variety of tests are needed to determine the appropriate diagnosis. Children suffering from juvenile arthritis have to ascertain the presence of the disease for over a month before it can be correctly identified.

The main problem that this condition causes in most families is frustration. Arthritis is supposed to affect only older people and so when a child is diagnosed with the condition, they are often confused and they do not know what to do.

If anything the condition is worse for children than it is for adults as they cannot always express the pain that they are in and it can be confusing for them why they are in so much pain all of the time.

Many people do mistake Juvenile Arthritis with the term 'Growing Pains' and while some pain and discomfort is to be expected throughout childhood, the pain should never be severe enough for it to cause any problems.

So, if your child is telling you that they are in a lot of pain, or if they look to be in a lot of pain with their joints when they are moving around, you should take them to see a physician right away.

Juvenile Arthritis varies in severity from child to child and so various tests will need to be carried out in order to determine how badly your child is suffering from it.

If you do suspect that your child could have Juvenile Arthritis, it is important that you take them to your local physician in order to be sure. Once there, the physician will run a few tests just to determine what the problem actually is.

The main thing that the physician will look for is whether the pain could be caused by a systemic disease. It can often be hard to diagnose Juvenile Arthritis and so that is why so many tests are needed to be done. Changes in lifestyle will be looked at such as if there has been a dramatic change in activity and also things such as whether the child has become ill with any form of fever should be consideres also.

A physical examination will be given on the affected areas and around those affected areas, just to have a better idea of how bad the problem is. As well as a physical test, tests such as Radiography and a blood count test may also be done.

Generally the amount of testing that is involved can be distressing for the child but it does need to be done just to be sure that the problem is Arthritis and nothing else.

The symptoms of Juvenile Arthritis can differ, but mainly they include some illness such as fever. The child will go through periods where they feel fine and then they will suddenly come down with an illness again. So if your child is frequently becoming ill and if they are in pain, then it is likely that they are suffering with Juvenile Arthritis.

Treatments Available For Children with Juvenile Arthritis The treatments that are available for children with Juvenile Arthritis include drugs, physiotherapy and occupational Therapy.

It really depends upon the severity of the condition as to which treatments your child will be given. One thing that you should remember, however, is that often the pain relief which is available to adults with Arthritis is not usually appropriate for children. Therefore when it comes to pain relief, it can sometimes be a little difficult to help your child to deal with it.

The treatment that is given to children is aimed to help them to move their joints more freely and to reduce the amount of paint hat they do have. Occupational Therapy is used to help the child to live better with their condition. That includes showing how improvements and changes can be made in everyday living in order to help to reduce the risk of any severe pain. It also allows them to live as independently as possible.

Physiotherapy is the main treatment that helps to reduce the pain and help movement of the joints that are affected. Ice packs or heat packs are given and gentle exercises are also incorporated to ensure that the joints do not become too stiff.

Stretches and Hydrotherapy are often used during Physiotherapy and many parents find that they really help their children to move a lot better and more freely.

Finally, drugs are often used to both reduce the inflammation of the joints and to reduce the amount of paint that the child is in. However, as mentioned earlier, some drugs are not suitable for children and so it is always worth checking with a doctor what you can and cannot give your child to control the pain.

Generally Ibuprofen is a good choice of pain relief, but again check with your doctor beforehand in order to see that it is suitable for your child.

Juvenile Arthritis can be really painful and restricting for a child and it is a condition which is not fully understood by parents throughout the world. There is treatment for it, but you first need to ensure that your child undergoes various tests by a physician, in order to diagnose the condition properly. Only then can you really start to use various treatments for your child and they should be given by a doctor.

Psoriatic arthritis

Five percent of people with psoriasis (a chronic skin disorder) are affected by psoriatic arthritis. Like rheumatoid arthritis, the joints, and in some cases the spine, are subjected to inflammation.

Psoriatic arthritis is a particular type of inflammatory arthritis that affects roughly twenty percent of those suffering from the chronic skin condition called Psoriasis. Psoriatic arthritis occurs much more frequently among those that have a particular tissue type. The tissue type most affected by psoriatic arthritis is HLA-B27.

For the most part, treatment of psoriatic arthritis is quite similar to treatment of rheumatoid arthritis. Mostly treatment involves treating patients with anti-inflammatory drugs, though I believe that an advantage to natural medicine therapies are that the same relief is effected, yet that a deeper cause is more fully addressed as well.

For example, rubbing emu oil or CBD hemp oil into the affected areas, brings ant-inflammatory medicine directly to the affected areas, particularly where the joints do not lie very deep beneath the skin's surface.

It has been shown that a combination of emu oil applied topically, along with nutritional supplements of glucosamine, chondroitin and/or MSM, can keep arthritis very much under some semblance of control.

One of the more unique characteristics of psoriatic arthritis is that about eighty percent of those suffering with psoriatic arthritis will develop psoriatic nail lesions which are known by pitting of the nails, or even the complete lack of a nail. When a person loses a whole nail, this is called onycholysis.

Of course onycholysis is a very general term meaning simply disease of deformity of the nail. These can include everything from ingrown toenails to all kinds of odd and rare nail fungus and other deformities of the nails.

Psoriatic arthritis can develop at any age, yet the average age that psoriatic arthritis usually appears is about ten years after the first signs of psoriasis. For most people with psoriatic arthritis, this condition makes an onset between the ages of thirty and fifty, yet it can occur in children and those of other ages as well.

Women and men seem to be pretty equally affected by psoriatic arthritis, whereas osteoarthritis affects nearly twice as many women as it does men. One in seven cases of psoriatic arthritis involve the arthritic symptoms occurring much earlier than any skin problems or skin involvement of the condition.

There are some different types of psoriatic arthritis. There is symmetric psoriatic arthritis where joints on both sides of the body are affected simultaneously. This type accounts for about fifty percent of all psoriatic arthritis cases.

Asymmetric psoriatic arthritis affects around thirty-five percent of people suffering from the disorder. This type of psoriatic arthritis tends to be more mild and does not occur in the same joints on both sides of the body.

Less than five percent of psoriatic arthritis patients suffer from arthritis mutilans which is characterized by severe joint damage and is known to progress over months and years until some type of severe damage is noticed.

Spondylitis is a type of psoriatic arthritis characterized by stiffness in the neck or spine and can also affect the feet or hands. Distal interphalangeal predominant arthritis is characterized by pain and stiffness in joints located closest to the tips of fingers and toes.

The main treatment used for psoriatic arthritis is the administering of anti-inflammatory drugs and nutitional supplements. When psoriatic arthritis does not respond to such treatment, sometimes immunosuppresants such as methotrexate may be used to treat the psoriasis in addition to the arthritis.

Fibromyalgia

Muscular pain, tingling, burning, and numbness are common symptoms of a repetitive strain injury. However, these symptoms are also common in a condition called Fibromyalgia.

Fibromyalgia basically means pain in the muscles, tendons and ligaments. It affects mostly women and up to 4% of the general population.

The pain of fibromyalgia occurs in areas where the muscles attach to bone or ligaments and is similar to the pain of arthritis.

The joints themselves are not affected, however, so they are not deformed nor do they deteriorate as they may in arthritic conditions. The pain typically originates in one area, usually the neck and shoulders, and then radiates out. Most patients report feeling some pain all the time; and many describe it as "exhausting." The pain can vary, depending on the time of day, weather changes, physical activity, and the presence of stressful situations; it has been described as stiffness, burning, stabbing, sudden, radiating, and aching. The pain is often more intense after disturbed sleep.

The other major complaint is fatigue, which some patients report as being more debilitating than the pain. Fatigue and sleep disturbances are, in fact, almost universal in patients with fibromyalgia, due to lack of serotonin, and if these symptoms are not present, then some experts believe that physicians should seek a diagnosis other than fibromyalgia.

Up to a third of patients experience depression, and disturbances in mood and concentration are very common.

Fibromyalgia patients are also prone to tension or migraine headaches. Other symptoms include dizziness, tingling or numbness in the hands and feet, and gastrointestinal problems, including irritable bowel syndrome with gas and alternating diarrhea and constipation. Some patients complain of urinary frequency caused by bladder spasms. Women may have painful menstrual periods.

Several years ago Fibromyalgia was a disability categorized as "psychological". It's hard to understand how it feels to be told you are mentally having a problem when your body will not perform what you are asking it to do. How can that possibly be mental?

Patients were, in effect, being told it was "all in your head".

Fortunately, the medical field has produced enough research to re-classify it as a true physical disability that is often paired with studies and treatments for arthritis and rheumatism.

People with FMS have the additional stress and frustration in their lives of trying to explain (all the time) why today they can do almost anything and the next day they can barely get out of bed.

Depression is a frequent side-effect of FMS and who can question it? Living with a body-wide toothache-like pain constantly is something only fellow sufferers can truly understand.

When we have "bad days" the pain can feel like there are hot curling irons jammed into our muscles. Can you even imagine that? Also imagine the fatigue of your muscles being so bad that it feels like they have turned to Jell-O. And no matter how much you try to exercise your muscles never feel normal again. It's always like battling Jell-O to make your body perform.

Spouses, family and others in your life have a hard time figuring out how you feel when you have FMS or chronic fatigue syndrome. There are times when you were accused of not pulling your own weight, or just plain sand bagging it. Many are accused of wanting extra attention.

After a while the Fibromyalgic doesn't like talking about it and they sure don't care for having to make excuses (can't go to a restaurant (Irritable Bowel Syndrome), can't go hiking; horseback riding; to the fairgrounds; the park and so on - while SOMETIMES the Fibromyalgic can't be stopped!). This is why I strongly recommend support groups where you can feel that you are not alone in this condition.

There is simply no way for anyone to understand what is going on internally with the Fibromyalgic body. Because you look absolutely normal, yet you feel like you will never perform normally again.

No one can see what the problem is. And since it is not such a known illness such as cancer it does not get the respect that people with cancer would get. No one would question a cancer patient about his or her illness because everyone has heard of it.

If you have bad days because of your illness with cancer no one would question it. But because Fibromyalgia has not been classified as a disease or given notoriety (such as a famous person getting FMS) it is relatively unknown.

As for doctors - it's very, common to end up with a FM diagnosis only after everything else is ruled out. Many people I've counseled with who have FMS also have now or have once had other problems such as herniated disks, degenerative disk disease, spontaneously fractured vertebrae or other bones, etc. that is why a Chiropractor is invaluable in treating Fibromyalgia.

FMS is NOT known to cause these problems or to be caused by these problems. It's just not rare to find such combination irregularities. FMS is often brought on (not caused by, but 'triggered' so to speak) by a trauma such as an accident/fall which causes what could be relatively minor physical pain, or major (doesn't really matter); even childbirth can 'trigger' it or any number of other things.

Any illness that comes on suddenly seems to trigger Fibromyalgia if the person is genetically inclined toward this syndrome.

Fibromyalagia can even cripple a person like arthritis or even Multiple Sclerosis, its symptoms AND the feeling is very much the same! More and more cases are being reported of people who are becoming bedridden, having to use Walkers or wheelchairs due to Fibromyalagia.

Chronic Fatigue, Depression, Chronic Pain/Myofascial Pain Syndrome are frequently found along with the FMS.

It can get so bad that being hugged (a breeze!) can be painful! A cat on a lap can feel like bone grinding against bone. Your socks touching your toes can be a nightmare of pain. Your sheets and blankets touching your toes or legs can be so painful you are unable to sleep. Elastic touching you anywhere is pure hell.

Imagine having even your clothes touching you your worst pain. It was so bad for one woman in her 30's, with small children (and a husband) that she used Dr. Kevorkian to end her misery. Some symptoms includes:

- Chronic pain throughout the body
- Burning, numbness and tingling

- Tenderness when pressure is placed on or around the neck, elbows, hips, thighs and knees.

- Sleep disorders

- Chronic fatigue or exhaustion

- Depression

- Anxiety

- Facial Pain

- Jaw Pain (TMJ)

- Memory Loss

- Irritable Bowel

- Tension or Migraine Headaches

- High sensitivity to foods and medications (allergic type reaction).

- Minimal tolerance to heat and cold

- High sensitivity to bright lights and sounds

- Hair Loss

Because symptoms develop gradually, this disease is often misdiagnosed. It is often diagnosed as a repetitive strain injury; sleep disorder condition, irritable bowel syndrome, rheumatoid arthritis or any other type of medical problem.

Based on the American College of Rheumatology a person is diagnosed with Fibromylagia when he or she suffers pain throughout the body for at least three months and has 11 out of 18 tender points present.

Experts estimate that 5 million to 8 million Americans have Fibromyalgia. Of these, 85 percent are women. One of the main risk factors is being a woman between the age of 30 and 60. Another risk factor is having a rheumatic disease, such as rheumatoid arthritis, lupus or Sjogren's syndrome.

Fibromyalgia also seems to run in families, so a gene may be at least partly responsible for the condition. Most people with fibromyalgia begin to notice symptoms between the ages of 20 and 40. But children and older adults may develop the condition. Women with fibromyalgia typically feel pain throughout their body.

Gout

Another painful type of arthritis is Gout. This form of the disease is characterized by unexpected bursts of intense pain, soreness, warmth and reddening of the affected areas, and joint swelling, particularly in the big toe. Gout is believed to be the result of excess uric acid crystals which are leached out of the blood and settle within the joint.

It is caused by the buildup of uric acid forming crystals of monosodium urate that are deposited on the articular cartilage of joints, tendons and surrounding tissues.

The crystals cause severe inflammation and pain in the joints and usually affect one joint at a time. If the condition remains untreated, the crystals will give rise to tophi, which can cause severe damage to the tissue.

The combination of high concentrations of uric acid or hyperuricemia and acidity in the blood stream is the precursor of gout arthritis. However, if taken separately, their incidence is not sufficient enough to cause gout.

The large toe is the main target of gout. However, it can also affect other joints in the leg, particularly the knee, ankle, and foot. In some severe cases, joints in the arm, including the hands, wrists, fingers, and elbows are also affected by gout.

This disease was once known to be a disease of the rich and the famous. It was attributed to excessive consumption of rich food and wine. Although diet is a causative agent, it is not the main cause of the condition.

This medical condition is a result of abnormal deposits of uric crystals in the joint cartilage. These crystals are later introduced into the synovial fluid.

However, not all persons with high concentration of uric acid will develop gout. This is dependent on the ability of the kidney to rid of the body of uric acid. This medical condition points to the heredity factor which explains partly why certain individual are predisposed to this medical condition.

This joint problem is defined as either primary, including idiopathic, or secondary, or complication, to another medical condition. Persons who consume high amounts of protein rich foods develop high levels of uric acid.

Excessive intake of alcohol also results to elevated concentrations of uric acid. Hereditary factors, like inborn errors of purine-pyrimidine metabolism, make one predisposed to gout. Individuals who are obese, diabetic and hypertensive are also suffering from gout. This is the reason why it is generally seen as a disease of the affluent societies.

This joint problem can be a complication of other diseases like metabolic syndrome and leukemia. The secondary gout can also be a co-morbidity of other diseases including polycythaemia, obesity, diabetes, and hypertension.

A patient with gout arthritis experiences excruciating pain, unexpected and burning pain, accompanied by swelling, redness and stiffness in the affected joint.

Men are usually more vulnerable than women especially in the large toe but it can also appear in other parts of their body. In some severe cases, the attack is accompanied by a low grade fever.

Contrary to common understanding, there is no cure for gout. What we are trying to treat and manage are the symptoms which can leave us debilitated when we suffer severe attacks.

The medical treatment has three objectives:

- Manage the symptoms
- Prevent attacks
- Reduce uric acid levels in the blood.

Pseudogout

Pseudogout is a disease which is often mistaken for the gout which is a sort of metabolic arthritis. Pseudogout is also a type of arthritis but it is not gout though the symptoms and the treatments of the gout and the pseudogout are almost of the similar types.

Pseudogout is a type of arthritis or inflammation caused because of the buildup of the Calcium Pyrophosphate Dihydrate crystals in the body.

Like the gout, in pseudogout also affects the large joint areas. The affected areas become red, swollen and stiff. Warmth is felt when touched. The attack of the pseudogout can last for a few days just like the gout attack.

In almost 75 percent of the gout case, the primary affected area is the big toe but in pseudogout the affected areas are the large joints areas of legs and arms. Gout is caused by the accumulation of the high uric acid crystals in the body while the pseudogout is caused by the accumulation of the Calcium Pyrophosphate Dihydrate crystals.

As earlier said the treatment of the pseudogout is similar to the treatment of the gout. In treating the pseudogout the main focus is remained on relieving the pain in the joint areas. Several types of non-steroid and anti-inflammatory medicines are used to reduce the extreme pain that felt in the joint areas.

NSAIDs drugs like the Ibuprofen or the Motrin and Advil, Aleve and Indocin are used primarily to treat the disease.

But using the NSAIDs drugs cannot be without some side effects. Some severe side effects like the stomach bleeding, hypertension and kidney malfunction can be occurred with the medicines. This is the reason why the patients of the pseudogout should always consult to the doctors before they go for using any medicine.

The patients should know about the side effects that can happen to most of the common adults after using the NSAIDs drugs.

Colchicine is another medication that the doctors prescribe to the patients who are not suited for the NSAIDs drugs. The drug helps in alleviating the pain, swelling and the tenderness of the skin. But it can also cause some side effects like vomiting, diarrhoea and stoamch pain. Sometimes bleeding can also occur.

Joint Injection is another popular treatment for the pseudogout. In this type of treatment the doctor will inject the injection to take out some joint fluid. The doctor then injects corticosteroid to reduce the pain and inflammation. There after anesthetic can be injected into the affected joints to numb the ailing joints.

Hemochromatosis or joint trauma due to the iron overload can be the reason for some of the pseudogout cases. In such cases the doctors try to treat the problem of hemochromatosis to treat the pseudogout.

Proper resting is important for the pseudgout patients. Proper resting helps in relieving the pain and swelling. The doctor must prescribe the patients to limit the daily activities.

You should keep in mind that the problem of the pseudogout can be prevented and controlled as long as the doctor finds out the suitable medications for you. If you are suffering from pseudogout then you must consult your doctor about the proper medication and food diet plans.

Scleroderma

Hardening and thickening of the surrounding skin characterizes Scleroderma, a disorder affecting the connective tissues of the body. Two types of this disease, both the localized and generalized forms, also impair other parts of the body like the:

- blood vessels
- joints
- internal organs

Doctors know that there are no similar or identical cases of scleroderma. Each case of the disease is different, making it necessary for your doctors to identify your disease subtype, stage, as well as the number of organs involved. This will help your doctor customize a specific scleroderma treatment that will help cure your disease

The treatment must address 4 key features of the disease which are the stages of inflammation, severity of autoimmunity, presence of vascular disease, and degree of tissue fibrosis.

Anti-inflammatory medications for scleroderma treatment address two types of inflammation. The first type is inflammation of the joints (arthritis), muscles (myositis), lining of the heart (pericarditis), or lining of the lung (pleuritis).

Sesositis is a collective term used if both pericarditis and pleuritis are present. Commonly used drugs for this stage of the disease are NSAID's such as ibuprofen. Corticosteroids such as prednisone are also used if NSAID's are not effective. Unfortunately, not all inflammatory phases of scleraderma respond to this therapy.

Skin inflammation and other tissue injury caused by scleroderma are not relieved by anti-inflammatory medications.

Immunosuppressive therapy is employed to limit the progression of the inflammatory phase of scleroderma. You immune system must be suppressed as its hyperactivity is causing the damaging inflammatory process.

Methotrexate, antithymocyte globulin, cyclosporine, mycophenolate mofetil have been studied as scleroderma treatment. So far, studies have showed that methotrexate did not produce any significant changes in skin inflammation.

Cyclosporine studies are limited due to the presence of renal toxicity. Mycophenolate mofetil or cyclophosphamide are the only drugs that show promising results.

Vascular changes of scleroderma are also treated with several drugs. Calcium channel blockers such as nefedipine help dilate the blood vessels to prevent or cure Raynaud's phenomenon, as well as reduce the incidence of digital ulcers.

These drugs also help improve blood flow to the skin and heart. ACE (angiotensin converting enzyme) inhibitors also help fix vasospasm in renal crisis of scleroderma. Blood circulation to the lungs is improved with the use of bosentan (endothelin-1 receptor inhibitor or epoprostenol (prostacyclin).

Anti-fibrotic agents are used to address the presence of excess collagen production in the skin and other organs affected by scleroderma. This scleroderma treatment acts by reducing the collagen production or destabilize tissue collagen.

These medications include colchicines, dimethyl sulfoxide, para-aminobenzoic acid (PABA). Not all medical experts advocate the use of these drugs as they give very little change in the collagen production. Some doctors prescribe D-penicillamine as an alternative.

Research is still being conducted to find the right medication for scleroderma treatment. So far, no universal drug is known to treat all signs and symptoms of scleroderma.

Lupus / systemic lupus erythematosus

Another autoimmune disease, Systemic lupus erythematosus causes anaemia, arthritis, chronic tiredness, fever, hair loss, kidney complications, mouth ulcers and skin eruptions.

Nearly 90 percent of sufferers are women, particularly those of childbearing age. However, children and older adults can also contract the disease. Lupus affects the:

- blood vessels
- heart
- joints
- kidneys
- nervous system
- internal organs
- surrounding skin

A lupus diagnosis typically doesn't appear in a patient's chart until after several years of battling painful symptoms that "might be" "could be" "though it was" a different disease.

Lupus is a sneaky disease, often hiding itself within the body and resisting any form of treatment or diagnosis until well into the disease's development.

Treatment options for Lupus have come a long way in the past ten years. There was a time when a systemic lupus diagnosis came with a three year life expectancy. Today, lupus is not expected to end in termination of life, but living with the chronic pain and the difficulties are tremendously difficult and even terrifying.

Lupus is a sneaky disease, traveling from one part of the body to another seeking out "enemy intruders" that are nothing more than normal bodily organs. A confused immune system can do a lot of damage, and learning to cope with the inconsistent and blind siding pain is a daily struggle.

Lupus is often misdiagnosed as osteoarthritis or rheumatoid arthritis. Unfortunately, treating lupus as any other disease doesn't alleviate any of the painful symptoms nor does it cease the damage the body is doing to itself.

Treating lupus is a chronic challenge for any physician. Because the disease won't "stand still," doctors constantly have to alter treatment courses in order to catch up with the disease.

A patient can effectively manage their symptoms and their pain for six months only to be struck out of the blue by another flare up at a different location throughout the body. This presents numerous challenges both for the patient and the physician.

NSAIDS pain relievers are often used to treat lupus discomfort. In some cases they work well and in other cases they simply aren't very effective. Just because one treatment option works well for a while, patients should be open to trying new treatment options if they begin to have difficulties down the road. After all, with such a slick disease, staying flexible and open to possibilities is the only way to manage the alterations in the body's general health.

Immunosuppressant medications and Biologics are along the first line of defense. While immunosuppressant medications do not necessarily treat pain, they do help to alleviate attacks which in turn alleviate painful symptoms.

Corticosteroids may be prescribed to help quite the inflammation that coincides with lupus. Inflammation can cause just as much pain as any other pain source.

When an organ is inflamed, it is highly irritated, to the point that normal functioning adds to the discomfort. For instance, an inflamed finger is going to look swollen, red, and it is going to be a constant source of pain for the body it is attached to.

Inflammation also makes the finger sensitive to other touch, even touch that normally feels good. This is what is going on inside the body when an organ becomes inflamed. Inflammation is not usually given enough credit for being a legitimate pain source.

While medications can be an effective form of pain control, they also have their own risks, especially their regular use. Only the patient and a competent physician can determine whether the risks of the chronic use of medications are worth the benefits. After all, lupus is a disease with the potential to be degenerative, and it is vital that a person afflicted with lupus is able to maintain a standard of health that can combat the illness.

Chronic corticosteroids can cause all types of damage, not to mention weight gain, facial puffiness, and even anger problems in sensitive patients. The use if chronic NSAID pain relievers also host a degree of risk including organ damage.

While immunosuppressant medications are effective at keeping lupus under control, the obvious effect of this medication is a depleted immune system.

Patients and physicians alike need to keep in mind that an emotional state does contribute to the degree of health a patient may experience. While anger is normal when diagnosed with a potentially fatal disease, anger can also inhibit the patient's ability to control their pain. There are numerous clinical studies which confirm that pain can be enhanced from chronic and extreme negative emotions.

This in no way implies that the pain is in the patient's head. It's not. It is very real with a physiological cause. It implies that pain is harder to manage when a patient is depressed.

Depression and anger are normal, but part of learning to cope with the chronic pain is also learning to recognize the psychological impact the pain has on a patient and the patient's life. When a patient can learn to recognize their emotional needs, their physical needs are easier to treat.

Patients who have experienced many pain relieving options and have experimented with numerous alternative therapies do report that alternative pain relief therapies can be somewhat effective. Lupus patients who have tried both acupuncture and massage therapies aimed at pain relief have stated that their results often surprised them.

One patient may respond better to alternative therapies because these techniques are quite personal and often help one pain over another, but when living with chronic pain a patient does get to the point that they are willing to try anything to alleviate it. In all fairness, a patient would accept a bottle of magic potion without question as long as it worked.

Carpal tunnel syndrome

Carpal tunnel syndrome reached epidemic proportions in the 90's and has now achieved a status equaling pandemic proportions in the 21st century.

With so much attention and hype the past 10-years concerning carpal tunnel syndrome in the workplace, you would think that a clear-cut picture would exist regarding the "how's" "why's" and "what is it's" of carpal tunnel.

Although carpal tunnel syndrome should be easily recognizable with such extensive media exposure, you would be amazed at how many people, including a lot of doctors, who do not recognize the symptoms or misdiagnose it as something other than carpal tunnel syndrome.

In order to provide a more clear picture of what carpal tunnel is, why and how it develops and what can be done to eliminate it, I have provided information below to explain the process so that you can better identify and therefore prevent carpal tunnel syndrome from taking over your life.

The carpal tunnel is a passageway in which the nine flexor tendons, median nerve, arteries, blood and lymphatic vessels pass through in order to supply function and movement to the fingers and wrist.

The carpal bones line the carpal tunnel on the posterior surface (backside) of the wrist with the transverse carpal ligament positioned on the anterior (front side) of the wrist.

The size of the carpal tunnel is about the size of the index finger in diameter, and the flexor tendons, arteries and nerves glide past one another with ease in a carpal tunnel that has not decreased in size.

Because the finger and wrist muscles are constantly overused in one-way movement patterns, (Gripping, squeezing, typing, etc.) a "muscle imbalance" develops, causing the carpal bones to shift, in turn, making the carpal tunnel smaller and impinging the structures within, resulting in painful and debilitating symptoms.

Symptoms include:

- Tingling
- Numbness
- Paresthesia (Pins & needles)
- Loss of grip-strength / coordination

Sensations involving tightness, discomfort, stiffness and pain on the front side of the hand and wrist may be present in carpal tunnel, but may also be symptoms of a general repetitive strain injury.

The only true telltale signs of carpal tunnel syndrome that you need to be aware of affect the thumb, index, middle and sometimes one-half of the ring finger. (All of the fingers and symptoms listed do not have to be experienced simultaneously for you to have carpal tunnel syndrome.)

If you have symptoms in your entire ring and/or little finger and your doctor tells you that you have carpal tunnel syndrome, you don't! The ULNAR nerve supplies function to the ring and little finger and has nothing to so with carpal tunnel syndrome. (If the ring and/or little fingers are affected, it may either be Cubital Tunnel Syndrome or Guyon's Syndrome)

Carpal tunnel syndrome can quickly and easily be eliminated by performing a good stretch and exercise program that addresses the existing muscle imbalance that is the cause of carpal tunnel in most cases.

Ankylosing spondylitis

The most frequent symptom of AS is one a lot of folks are intimate with, lower back pain and/or stiffness. This sign can come out as soon as adolescence that causes numerous individuals with ankylosing spondylitis to be misdiagnosed as teenagers with a sports related injury.

The stiffness and pain are often slow, which indicates many people do not inform their physician about the pain. The stiffness and pain are produced by the inflammation in the spine, that if not remedied, can bring about a fusing of the vertebrae or ankylosis.

When this occurs, the pain vanishes, but so does the mobility in the spine. The ankylosis can bring about a frontward curvature of the chest region, that diminishes breathing ability. The fusion can additionally go on to the rib cage, triggering ribs to fuse to the spine, diminishing lung function. Further symptoms of AS are arthritis in other joints (usually the knees, hips, and ankles) and inflammation of the cartilage adjacent to the eyes, breast bone, the heart, and kidneys.

An accurate identification of AS can be tough to obtain. Initial warning signs can frequently be created by other, more ordinary diseases. It's particularly tricky to identify in women since they typically have less implication of the spine, commonly but not always.

Someone may be required to suffer with the pain for quite a few years before ankylosing spondylitis is ever thought about. The analysis for AS are essentially very straightforward.

They comprise the customary physical exam and medical history, then the physician will arrange an x-ray of the spine and a blood test for the HLA-B27 marker. The physical assessment may demonstrate initial symptoms such as restricted mobility of the spine, diminished breathing capability, and eye inflammation. The spine x-ray will demonstrate if fusion of the vertebrae has already happened. When accurately identified, therapy starts.

Therapy consists of physical therapy, the taking of non-steroid anti-inflammatory drugs (NSAIDs), and then increased exercise. The NSAIDs decrease the pain and inflammation of the involved joints, which can help mobility. In people where other joints, like the hips, knees, and ankles, are inflamed, the NSAIDs might not work acceptably.

If that is the case, there are more drugs that can be utilized such as methotrexate and sulfasalazine. Methotrexate is more successful than sulfasalazine, however it's possibly poisonous to bone marrow and the liver. Patients having methotrexate therapy have to have regular blood tests to find out if any of those organs are being injured.

Through enhanced mobility comes the exercise and physical therapy to recover posture and boost mobility and breathing capability. Every exercise regimen must be endorsed by a physician so the patient doesn't inadvertently hurt him/herself.

Ankylosing spondylitis typically involves the joints of the spine, although it can also involve other joints, particularly the hips. AS may also intermittently produce inflammation of the chest wall, eyes, lungs, and heart.

If the inflammation doesn't get cared for, it can ultimately lead to permanent damage and scarring. A few individuals have a minor variety of this disease, others are unlucky enough to experience the destructive type.

This disease might or might not get worse, according to a number of things. These things involve, your age when the disease started, which joints are involved, and how soon you received an accurate diagnosis.

Physicians aren't certain of the trigger for AS, but they do understand that genetics has a role in the disease. About 95% of patients identified with this disease possess a gene that manufactures a genetic marker, HLA-B27.

Still, possessing this gene doesn't mean someone is certain to acquire the disease. There's barely a 40% possibility of acquiring AS if you have the gene. Furthermore, you don't have to possess this gene to acquire AS.

This chronic inflammatory condition of the spine can cause fusion of the vertebrae, resulting in rigidity of the spinal column. The disease starts by settling into the tissue surrounding the joint, causing lingering stiffness and pain in the lower back.

Medical science has yet to discover the exact cause of this disease, which affects other joints in addition to the spine. It has been noted, however, that spondylitis sufferers all have HLA-B27, a genetic marker setting apart people who have the highest risk of acquiring the disorder. Men aged between 16 to 35 are the ones usually affected, although the disease can also strike women.

Bursitis / tendonitis

These types of arthritis are recognized by their chiefly inflammatory symptoms. Bursitis is characterized by inflamed bursa sacs, fluid-filled sacs that help muscles and tendons move smoothly across the bones.

Tendonitis, or tendinitis is an inflammation of the tendons, connective elastic tissue found between the bones and muscles. The tendon sheath is also susceptible to inflammation, leading to a disorder known as tenosynovitis. In all cases, the inflammation results in stiff and painful movement.

Bursitis is unpleasant inflammation or irritation of the bursa. The bursa is a soft sac filled with fluid that covers and pads the movement between bones, tendons and muscles near joints. Bursitis can happen due to an injury, infection, chronic overuse of a joint, trauma, rheumatoid arthritis, or gout.

For the symptoms, individuals in distress from bursitis usually feel discomfort and tenderness around the affected joint or tendon. The bursae sacs may swell making movement of the affected joint challenging. The joints most commonly impacted by bursitis are:

- shoulder
- elbow
- wrist
- hand
- knee
- foot

Infectious arthritis

Bacteria, virus and fungi are the culprits involved in Infectious arthritis. To diagnose this type of arthritis, culturing a tissue sample from the infected joint determines the existence of these microorganisms. Infectious arthritis comes in several forms, namely:

- Septic arthritis caused by a bacterial invasion.

- Tuberculous arthritis common in tuberculosis sufferers.

- Fungal arthritis stemming from fungal infection.

- Gonococcal arthritis occurring with those infected with gonorrhoea.

- Viral arthritis resulting from viral infections.

Lyme disease

Lyme disease is often caused by the bite of an infected deer tick. This disorder usually targets:

- eyes
- heart
- joints
- nervous system
- skin

Reactive arthritis

Also known as Reiter's syndrome, Reactive arthritis causes inflammation of the joints, particularly in the areas of ligament and tendon connection. Sufferers of this type of arthritis experience other illnesses like:

- cervicitis
- conjuctivitis
- cystitis
- skin sores
- prostatitis
- urethritis

Sjogren's syndrome

Sjorgren's Syndrome causes irregularity in the functions of the moisture-producing glands of the body, resulting in dryness in the salivary and lacrimal (tear-producing) glands. This disorder is also characterized by other physical indicators.

Sjogren's Syndrome is a strange name for a mysterious, little known, autoimmune illness. During the early 1900s it was first called "keratoconjunctivitis sicca" by Swedish ophthalmologist Henrik Sjogren. "Sicca" is the term used to describe dryness of the eyes (and mouth).

Sjogren's affects the "exocrine", or moisture producing, glands. Some people think it's just a "dry mouth" or "dry eyes", but it can affect the whole body in various ways. Sometimes symptoms are mild, and nothing more than an annoyance. Other times, symptoms are major, severely reduce the quality of life, and can lead to some pretty awful complications if not noticed and treated.

Women seem to get Sjogren's more often than men; in fact, 90% of Sjogren's patients are female, though there are a number of men who suffer from it too. It can take YEARS to receive a diagnosis of Sjogren's, and sometimes people go to numerous doctors before the proper diagnosis is finally made.

Blood tests, eye tests, and lip biopsies can help make a diagnosis of Sjogren's. Sometimes antibodies show up immediately in blood tests for Sjogren's. At other times, a person might still have Sjogren's, but the antibodies won't show up in blood tests until the disease has progressed further. In a few people, the antibodies don't show in blood tests at all.

In a lip biopsy, the inner lip is numbed and a sampling is taken from the saliva glands. The Shirmer test measures tear production in the eyes.

Osteoporosis

This degenerative bone disease leads to weak, brittle bones and loss of bone tissue, increasing the risk of breaks and fractures. It is a preventive non-symptomatic disorder creeps up slowly and becomes apparent in advanced age, particularly in women.

The disease which makes the bone more prone to fractures is known as osteoporosis and the name indicates porous bones.

The bone mineral density (BMD) reduces followed by deterioration of micro-architecture of bone and alteration of bone proteins. World Health Organization (WHO) defines that the bone mineral density in osteoporosis is less than 2.5 as measured by DXA. The disease may be classified as primary type 1, primary type 2 or secondary. Primary 1 or postmenopausal osteoporosis is very frequently noticed in women after the menopause. Primary 2 or senile osteoporosis is common after the age of 75 and is observed in both males and females in the ration of 2:1. Secondary osteoporosis can affect both men and women at any age in equal proportion.

This disease crops up due to prolonged use of glucocorticoids so also known as glucocoticoid-induced osteoporosis.

Lifestyle changes and sometimes medications can reduce the risk of this disease. Lifestyle changes comprise diet, exercise and fall-prevention. Fall-prevention includes exercise to tone deambulatory muscles, proprioception-improvement excercises and equilibrium therapies.

Exercise and its anabolic effect can reduce the risk as well as cure this disease. Medication involves calcium, vitamin D, bisphosphonates and others. This disease is actually a component of frailty syndrome.

Osteoporosis results in declination of strength of bones that makes them fragile. The bones become abnormally porous similar to the sponge. The skeleton weakens and is more prone to fractures. Osteopenia is a condition where the bones are slightly less dense than the normal bone but this dense feature is not comparable to that found in osteoporosis.

Protein, calcium and collagen are the chief constituents that are responsible for the strength of the bone. Bones that are affected by osteoporosis may break very easily after a very minor injury that in general cannot cause harm to the normal bone.

This break or fracture of the bone may be in the form of cracking or collapsing. Spine, hips, ribs and wrists are the major portions of body that are frequently affected by this disease and can be fractured by a minor dent.

The disease cannot be characterized by specific symptoms but the major noticeable sign is increased risk of fractures. Individuals suffering from this disorder generally encounter with fractures after a very minute injury which normal individuals generally do not face. These fractures are known as fragility fractures.

Fractures form the well identified symptom of osteoporosis. In older individuals these fractures result in devastating acute and chronic pain that results in further disability and even early mortality. The fractures may be asymptomatic and the symptoms of vertebral collapse are sudden back pain, radiculopathic pain and spinal cord compression. Multiple vertebral fractures result in stooped posture, loss of height, chronic pain and reduced mobility.

Fractures of the long bones often require surgery. Hip fracture requires prompt surgery and many serious risks are also associated with it particularly deep vein thrombosis, pulmonary embolism and increased mortality.

Fracture Risk Calculators consider a number of factors that are responsible for fractures and they are bone mineral density (BMD), age, smoking, alcohol usage, weight and gender. FRAX and Dubbo are the well known fracture risk calculators known in the present era.

Osteoporosis is also associated with the increased risk of falling and it causes fractures of hip, wrist and spine. The risk of falling is increased by impaired eyesight which may be due to glaucoma and macular degeneration.

Balance disorder, movement disorders, dementia and sarcopenia are other factors that also increase the risk of falling. Collapse may result due to cardiac arrhythmias, vasovagal syncope, orthostatic hypotension and seizures. Removal of hurdles from the environment can reduce the risk of falls.

The risk factors for osteoporotic fractures can be placed under the category of modifiable and non-modifiable ones.

Apart from these factors some diseases are also known that also result in this disorder and in some cases medication also increases the risk of osteoporosis.

Caffeine is not a risk factor for this disease. The most important risk factors for this disorder are increased age, female gender, and estrogen deficiency after menopause or oophorectomy that causes rapid declination of bone mineral density while in males reduction in testosterone levels can result in osteoporosis.

The individuals with family history of this disorder are at increased risk and the incidence is 25-80%. About 30 genes can be considered responsible for this disease and small stature can be responsible for osteoporosis.

A number of potentially modifiable factors can be considered responsible for osteoporosis for example excess usage of alcohol although lower doses of alcohol have a beneficial effect on human body.

Bone density starts increasing as the alcohol intake is increased. Chronic heavy drinking also causes increased risk of fractures. Vitamin D deficiency among old individuals is very common and this mild insufficiency of vitamin D is due to increased production of the parathyroid hormone (PTH).

Increased secretion of this hormone causes bone resorption that result in bone loss. Positive association has been noticed between serum 1, 25-dihydroxycholecalciferol levels and bone mineral density while PTH is negatively associated with bone mineral density.

Tobacco smoking is an independent factor for osteoporosis as it inhibits the activity of osteoblasts. Smoking also results in increased breakdown of exogenous estrogen, earlier menopause, lower body weight and all these factors result in lower bone density.

Research has shown that consumption of high protein diet also increases loss of calcium from the bones in the urine.

Nutrition plays an important role in maintenance of strong bones. Lower dietary calcium, phosphorus, zinc, magnesium, iron, fluoride, boron, copper, and vitamins A, E, K and C also cause lower bone density. Excess of sodium and high blood acidity have a negative effect on bones. Lower intake of proteins by older individuals also increases the risk of lower bone density.

Imbalance of omega 6 to omega 3 polyunsaturated fats is other risk factors. Underweight is another factor that causes this disease.

Excessive exercise also has a negative effect over bones as noticed in marathon runners later in their lives. In women heavy exercise results in decreases estrogen levels that increases the risk of osteoporosis. Heavy metals also play a very important part in occurrence of this disease.

A strong association has been found between cadmium, lead and bone disease. Low level exposure of cadmium results in increased loss of bone mineral density in both males and females causing increased risk of fractures which is more common in females. Higher cadmium exposure causes osteomalacia.

Some studies have indicated that excessive consumption of the soft drinks also increase the risk of osteoporosis.

Osteoporotic bone fractures cause considerable pain, reduced quality of life, lost workdays and disability. About 30% of the individuals that suffer from the hip fracture require long-term nursing care. Older individuals develop pneumonia followed by blood clots in the leg veins. These blood clots may later invade the lungs due to prolonged bed rest after the hip fracture. The risk of death of the patient also increases due to this disease.

About 20% of the women suffering from hip fracture die very early. A person suffering from spine fracture due to osteoporosis is at increased risk of experiencing another fracture in the near future.

About 20% of the postmenopausal women who suffer from the vertebral fracture are also at the risk of suffering from another vertebral fracture in the following years.

Osteoporosis is an important health issue. In the United States about 44 million individuals suffer from low bone density out of which the 55% of the individuals belong to the age of 50 or more. Lots of dollars are spent for the treatment of such individuals. One in two Caucasian women will suffer from fracture due to this disease in her lifetime.

About 20% of the individuals suffering from the hip fracture will die in the following year. About one-third of the individuals experiencing hip fracture are transferred to the nursing homes for long-term care. With increasing age the chances of this disease and the cases of fractures increase exponentially.

Bone density can be calculated by the total amount of bone present in the skeletal structure. Higher the bone density stronger is the bone. It is greatly influenced by the genetic factors which in turn are also affected by the environmental factors and medications.

Men have higher bone density as compared to the women and similarly African Americans have higher bone density than the Caucasian Americans.

The bone density starts accumulating during the childhood and reaches its peak at the age of 25 and can be maintained for about 10 years. Bone density starts depleting with the rate of 0.3-0.5% every year as a result of aging in both men and women after the age of 35.

Bone density is also maintained by the levels of estrogen in women. Bone density reduces after menopause as the estrogen levels start declining. During the first 5-10 years after menopause women experience reduction of bone density with the rate of 2-4%.

So about 20-30% of bone strength is lost during this period. The increased rate of loss of bone density in women after menopause is the major cause of osteoporosis in them and is also known as postmenopausal osteoporosis.

The National Osteoporosis Foundation has suggested that the individuals belonging to some specific groups must undergo dual energy X-ray absorptiometry (DEXA or DXA) and these include all postmenopausal women who are below 65 years of age and are at the risk of getting affected with osteoporosis.

All the women who are above 65 years of age and postmenopausal women with fractures must undergo this therapy. Women who are about to start the treatment for osteoporosis and those who have 50 medical conditions associated with osteoporosis must undergo dual energy X-ray absorptiometry.

A number of diseases and disorders have been found to be coupled with osteoporosis. For some of these diseases the mechanism that affects the bone metabolism is known while for others the mechanism is somewhat complex and not clearly understood.

In common terms immobilization results in bone loss for example, localized osteoporosis can occur after prolonged immobilization of a fractured limb. This condition has been frequently observed in the athletes.

Other examples of bone loss are space flight or people using wheel chairs due to some reasons. Hypogonadal states cause secondary osteoporosis and include Turner syndrome, Klinefelter syndrome, Kallman syndrome and anorexia nervosa.

In females hypogonadism crops up due to estrogen deficiency. It can appear as early menopause or from prolonged premenopausal amenorrhea. A bilateral oophorectomy or premature ovarian failure also causes declination of the estrogen levels. In males the deficiency of testosterone is responsible for secondary osteoporosis.

Endocrine disorders namely Cushing's syndrome, hyperparathyroidism, thyrotoxicosis, hypothyroidsm, diabetes mellitus type 1 and 2, acromegaly and adrenal insufficiency also cause osteoporosis.

Reversible bone loss has been noticed in pregnancy and lactation. Malnutrition, malabsorption and parenteral nutrition also cause this disease. Coeliac disease, Crohn's disease, lactose intolerance, surgery and severe liver disease and some other gastrointestinal disease can also be the root cause of osteoporosis. Inadequate uptake of calcium, vitamin D, vitamin K and vitamin B12 can also cause bone loss. Patients suffering from rheumatoid arthritis, ankylosing spondylitis and systemic lupus erythematosus combined with some systemic disorders like amyloidosis and sarcoidosis also result in osteoporosis.

Renal insufficiency can cause osteodystrophy. Hematologic disorders like multiple myeloma, monoclonal gammopathies, lymphoma, leukemia, sickle cell anemia and thalassemia can also cause osteoporosis.

Several inherited disorders like Marfan syndrome, osteogenesis imperfect, hemochromatosis, hypophosphatasia, glycogen storage diseases, Ehlers-Danlos syndrome and Gaucher's disease also result in bone loss. Parkinson's disease and chronic obstructive pulmonary disease also result in osteoporosis.

Certain medications are also found to be associated with the increased risk of osteoporosis and only steroids and anticonvulsants play a major role in this category.

Steroid induced osteoporosis (SIOP) which generally arises due to usage of glucocorticoids. Barbiturates, phenytoin and antiepileptic drugs also increase the metabolism of vitamin D resulting in bone loss. L-thyroxine taken for the cure of thyrotoxicosis also increases the risk of bone loss. Several drugs like aromatse inhibitors, methotrexate, certain anti-metabolite drugs and gonadotropin-releasing hormone agonists also cause bone loss.

Anticoagulants like heparin and warfarin also increase the risk of osteoporosis. Proton pump inhibitors interfere with the calcium absorption resulting in chronic phosphate binding that increases the risk of osteoporosis.

Chronic lithium therapy also causes osteoporosis. Imbalance between bone resorption and bone formation is the major mechanism underlying this disease. There is continuous remodeling of the bone matrix and 10% of the bone mass may undergo remodeling at any time.

This process of remodeling occurs in the bone multicellular units (BMU) that were first discovered by Frost in 1963. Bone is resorbed by the osteoclast cells that are derived from the bone marrow and after that new bone is deposited by the osteoblasts.

There are three major mechanisms which contribute in the development of osteoporosis. These include inadequate peak bone mass in which the skeleton develops insufficient mass and strength during growth, excessive bone resorption and inadequate formation of new bone during remodeling. All these mechanisms together contribute in the development of fragile bone tissue.

Hormonal factors strongly participate in bone resorption for example, estrogen deficiency increases bone resorption as well as decreases deposition of new bone which is a normal process in the weight-bearing bones.

The amount of estrogen required to suppress this process is generally lower than that needed for the stimulation of uterus and breast. The a-form of estrogen receptor seems to play an important role in bone turnover and calcium metabolism also plays an important role in this process.

Deficiency of calcium and vitamin D result in impaired bone formation and even the parathyroid glands react actively when the calcium level is low and secrete the parathyroid hormone that increases bone resorption.

Calcitonin secreted by the thyroid glands also participates in bone resorption but the role is not very clear.

Osteoclasts are activated by a number of molecular signals of which the best studied is RANKL. This molecule is produced by the osteoblasts and other cells namely the lymphocytes that together activate the RANK molecule. Osteoprotegerin (OPG) binds strongly to RANKL and results in increased bone resorption. RANKL, RANK and OPG are closely related to the tumor necrosis factor and its receptors.

Local production of eicosanoids and interleukin also play significant role in bone turnover and their excess or reduced production may play a positive role in development of osteoporosis.

Trabecular bone is the sponge-like bone that is present at the terminal portion of the long bones and the vertebrae. Cortical bone is the hard outer shell of bones and middle of the long bones.

As the osteoblasts and osteoclasts mark the surface of the bones the trabecular bone is subjected to turnover and remodeling and so the bone density decreases and the microarchitecture of bone also gets distorted. The weaker spicules of the trabecular bone are replaced by weak bones.

Hip, wrist and spine are at the higher risk of being fractures so they have higher trabecular to cortical bone ratio.

These areas of body rely on trabecular bone for strength and any imbalance in remodeling may result in degeneration of these areas. Loss of trabecular bone begins at the age of 35 and the process if 50% frequent in females and 30% in males.

Osteoporosis can be diagnosed by radiotherapy and by measuring the bone mineral density (BMD) and the most popular method for this is the dual energy X-ray abosorptiometry (DEXA).

Certain blood tests and even investigations associated with bone cancer can be performed. Conventional radiotherapy alone or in combination with MRI and CT scan is very effective for the diagnosis of osteopenia. A number of clinical decision rules have been made to predict the risk of fractures which are liable to occur in this disease.

The QFracture score was developed in 2009 which is based on age, BMI, smoking status, alcohol usage, rheumatoid arthritis, diabetes type 2, cardiovascular disease, corticosteroids, liver disease and history of falls in men.

In females, hormone replacement therapy, history of osteoporosis, menopausal symptoms and gastrointestinal malabsorption are taken into account.

The Dual energy X-ray absorptiometry is now-a-days considered as the most powerful tool for the diagnosis of this disease. Osteoporosis is generally diagnosed when the bone mineral density (BMD) is less than or equal to 2.5 and the values are generally indicated by using a T-score. World Health Organization (WHO) has set certain standards for the disease identification like if T-score is greater than 1.0 then the individual is normal, if it is between 1.0-2.5 then the person may have osteopenia and if it is less than 2.5 then the condition is identified as osteoporosis. Chemical biomarkers are the perfect tools for identifying bone degradation.

The enzyme cathepsin K carries out the breakdown of type 1 collagen protein and so is an important constituent in bones. Increased urinary excretion of C-telopeptides also serves as a biomarker for this disease.

Quantitative computer tomography gives a separate estimate of bone mineral density (BMD) for trabecular and cortical bones in mg/cm3.

This technique can be performed at both axial and peripheral sites, is sensitive to time, can analyze a region of any shape and size and excludes irrelevant tissues like fat and muscles but it also suffers from some drawbacks like it requires a high radiation dose, CT scanners are large and expensive and results are more dependent on individual operator.

Quantitative ultrasound can be performed for disease diagnosis as it has many advantages like modality is small, no ionizing radiation is required, results can be achieved very quickly with greater accuracy and the cost of the device is also very low.

Calcaneus is the most preferred skeletal site used while using this device. The US Preventive Services Task Force (USPSTF) in 2011 recommended that all the women who are of 65 years or more must be screened with bone densitometry as they are at increased risk of getting affected with osteoporosis.

Changes in the lifestyle can help to prevent the risks associated with osteoporosis. Tobacco smoking and inadequate alcohol intake are in general linked with this disease and if they are stopped then the risk may be minimized.

Balanced nutrition and proper exercise also delay bone degradation. Proper diet includes efficient intake of calcium and vitamin D.

People suffering from this disease are generally given Vitamin D tablets and calcium supplements especially biophosphonates.

Vitamin D supplements are alone not enough to prevent the risk of fractures so they are coupled with calcium supplement to minimize the risk. Calcium supplements are generally available in two forms namely calcium carbonate and calcium citrate.

Calcium carbonate is generally very cheap so selected my majority of individuals and is generally taken along with food while calcium citrate is expensive, more effective and can be taken without food.

Patients taking H2 blockers or proton pump inhibitors are suggested to take calcium citrate as they are not able to absorb calcium carbonate. In patients with renal disease, more active forms of vitamin D like cholecalciferol are recommended as kidney is unable to generate calcitriol from calcidiol which is the storage form of vitamin D. Vitamin D3 supplements are generally recommended by the doctors.

Intake of high dietary proteins is associated with increased excretion of calcium in urine so the risk of fractures is increased. Studies indicate that protein is essential for calcium absorption but excessive protein inhibits this process.

Estrogen Hormone therapy after the menopause has shown positive results in preventing bone loss, increase bone loss and risk of fractures. It is helpful in preventing fractures in postmenopausal women. Estrogen can be taken orally or as a skin patch.

It is also available in combination with progesterone and can be taken orally of as skin patch. Progesterone along with estrogen reduces the risk of uterine cancer.

Women who had undergone hyeterectomy can also take estrogen as they don't have the risk of uterine cancer. FDA has recommended the antiresorptive drugs to be the most effective agents against osteoporosis as they decrease the level of calcium loss from the bones. Biophosphonates are most effective antiresorptive agents as they reduce the risk of fractures especially those associated with hip, wrist and spine.

Fosamax, Actonel, Boniva and Reclast are the most popularly available biophosphonates. To reduce side effects all biophosphonates are taken orally generally 30 minutes before breakfast. Food, calcium supplements, iron tablets, vitamins, antacids reduce the absorption of oral biophosphonates and thereby reducing their effectiveness. Therefore, they must be taken orally in the morning only.

Calcitonin is a hormone that is approved by FDA to be used against osteoporosis. Calcitonins can be derived from a number of animal species but those obtained from salmon are most effect in preventing bone loss. Calcitonin injection can be given intravenously, subcutaneously or intransally.

Intranasal administration is the most effective method. This hormone is very effective in preventing bone loss in the postmenopausal women and also increases bone density along with strengthening of spine. It is a weaker antiresorptive agent than biophosphonates. It is not as effective as estrogen in increasing bone density and bone strengthening. It is also not very effective in preventing spine and hip fractures. For these drawbacks it is not the first choice of treatment for the women suffering from osteoporosis.

Vitamin K also plays an important role in stimulating collagen production, promoting bone health and reducing the risk of fracture. Vitamin K is of two types particularly vitamin K1 and K2.

K1 is found in the green leafy vegetables and K2 is found in various forms especially menaquinone-4 (MK4) and menaquinone-7(MK7). MK4 is most intensely researched by the researchers and is found to be effective in reducing the risks associated with fractures in osteoporosis.

MK4 is produced in testes, pancreas and arterial walls by the conversion of K1 in body. MK7 is not produced in human body but is converted in the intestine by the action of bacteria on K1.

MK4 and MK7 both are found in the dietary supplements given in United States for bone health. The

US FDA has not approved any form of vitamin K for treatment of this disease.

MK7 has not shown any effectiveness for reducing the risk of fractures. In clinical trials MK4 has shown positive results in reducing the risks associated with fractures and are used for treating the patients of this disease as it is approved by the Ministry of Health in Japan since 1995.

In Japan, the patients are given daily doses of MK4 with the quantity reaching up to 45 mg. About 87% reduction in risks associated with fractures have been noticed. MK4 has also reduced the risk of fractures caused by corticosteroids, anorexia nervosa, cirrhosis of liver, postmenopausal osteoporosis, Alzheimer's disease and Parkinson's disease in the clinical trials.

A number of studies have shown that aerobics, weigh bearing and resistance exercises can increase the bone mineral density in the postmenopausal women.

The Bone-Estrogen-Strength-Training (BEST) Project at the University of Arizona has identified six different weight bearing exercises that are helpful in maintaining the bone mineral density among the patients of osteoporosis.

One year of regular jumping has helped in increasing the bone mineral density as well as moment of inertia of the proximal tibia in the normal postmenopausal women.

Exercise combined with hormone replacement therapy has also shown positive results. In choosing the appropriate medication for a patient suffering from osteoporosis the physician checks all the aspects that are associated with the family background and also the seriousness of the disease.

If a postmenopausal woman suffers from hot flashes and vaginal dryness then hormone replacement therapy is the best option as it can prevent osteoporosis.

If prevention and treatment is the only option left in osteoporosis then doses of biophosphonates are given. Biophosphonates are best for treating postmenopausal women with this disease.

Calcitonin is a weaker antiresorptive agent than biophosphonates and is prescribed for the individuals who do not react to other medications.

Patients with moderate to severe osteoporosis effective biophosphonates are recommended. The long-term usage of corticosteroids can increase the risk of osteoporosis.

These substances decrease calcium absorption from the intestine, increase loss of calcium in urine from the kidneys, increase loss of calcium from bones. To reduce these risks patients are advised to have adequate intake of calcium and vitamin D.

Additional doses of other medicines along with calcium and vitamin D are also prescribed by the physicians. The American Medical Association (AMA) and other reputable medical associations recommend that repeat bone density testing should not be performed while monitoring osteoporosis treatment.

Patients with osteoporosis have high rate of mortality due to fractures which may be lethal. Hip fractures decrease mobility and increase the risk of additional complications like deep venous thrombosis and pneumonia.

The chances of hip fractures increase by 13.5% in patients with osteoporosis.Vertebral fractures however reduce the chances of death but increase other risks like chronic pain of neurogenic origin, multiple fractures can cause kyphosis associated with breathing impairment. Quality of life also gets reduced.

Other Forms of Rheumatic Diseases

- Avascular Necrosis - also recognized by the medical term, osteonecrosis
- Behcet's Disease - characterized by chronic inflammation.

- Complex Regional Pain Syndrome - CRPS, or reflex sympathetic dystrophy.

- Diffuse Idiopathic Skeletal Hyperostosis - causes calcification in the spinal disks.

- Inflammatory Bowel Disease - commonly accompanied by complications of arthritis and osteoporosis.

- Mixed Connective Tissue Diseases - a combination of several rheumatic diseases.

- Polymyalgia Rheumatica - caused by giant cell arteritis.

- Raynaud's Phenomenon - primarily affects the blood vessels, causing them to constrict.

- Vasculitides - a disease characterized by inflamed blood vessels.

CHAPTER 5: TREATMENTS

Modern treatments for arthritis

Modern medicine, unfortunately, has not found a cure for arthritis yet. Doctors do not even know exactly what causes arthritis. Modern treatments for arthritis can be divided into two categories - drugs and therapy.

Therapy encompasses traditional physical therapy and also occupational therapy. Physical therapy is a relatively old treatment for arthritis. It simply involves doing various exercises targeted at reducing the stiffness in the muscles and joints. This makes movement and physical activity somewhat easier and less painful.

This is important because many patients suffering from arthritis experience so much pain simply moving that they are rendered immobile.

Occupational therapy involves physical therapy coupled with training to perform useful tasks. This is also very important for arthritis patients, as they usually find themselves unemployed because of their inability to perform physical tasks. Some people are even bedridden by the disease. Occupational therapy is therefore a very important part of helping a patient learn to live with arthritis.

Modern drugs used to treat arthritis are generally only able to address the symptoms of arthritis. Drugs attempt to reduce the inflammation and swelling, but do not address the root cause of arthritis.

Natural treatments for arthritis

Turmeric and ginger extract has long been used in traditional medicine as a remedy for arthritis. They help to reduce the inflammation of joint tissues and the subsequent swelling.

Recent studies have found that this form of treatment is actually more effective than modern medicines. Turmeric and ginger extracts reduce arthritic swelling faster than modern drugs for arthritis do.

Using vitamins: Vitamin B3, also known as niacin, is another natural treatment for arthritis. It maintains the integrity of the tissues surrounding the joint. Arthritis generally causes damage in the form of cell destruction in the joints and muscles.

Vitamin B3 helps to counter this. Foods such as fish, poultry and red meats are rich in Vitamin B3. This makes it easy and natural to add Vitamin B3 to your daily food intake.

An extract from New Zealand's green-lipped mussel has been found to contain a glycoprotein which may help treat arthritis. The presence of this compound is thought to indirectly prevent the inflammation which occurs when the body's immune system starts attacking healthy tissue. The glycoprotein achieves this by blocking certain actions of neutrophils, the white blood cells which alert the immune system.

The element Manganese has also proven to be effective in the treatment of arthritis. It acts as a facilitator for the action of enzymes. It also retards the aging process.

Since the effect of arthritis on the joints is similar to that of aging, Manganese is effective at countering this.

Arthritis bracelets

One of the most controversial alternative treatments for this disease is arthritis bracelets. Arthritis bracelets contain permanent magnets inside them. These magnets produce static magnetic fields that can reportedly cure individuals from arthritis when placed in the right areas.

The effectiveness of arthritis bracelets are based on founding principles of magnet or magnetic therapy, also known as magnotherapy.

Studies have been conducted to determine the effectiveness of arthritis bracelets. These studies will typically divide subjects into three groups: one would wear arthritis bracelets using standard magnet strengths, another would wear arthritis bracelets using weak magnet strengths, while the last group would use arthritis bracelets using no magnets at all. All users would have to wear their bracelets for twelve weeks or a span of three months.

The results favored the use of arthritis bracelets. Firstly, the study was able to rule out any lasting influence of factors like the use of painkillers and personal beliefs of users on the effects of the magnetic therapy products.

Secondly, the study revealed that those who reported with the most favorable results came from the group wearing arthritis bracelets using standard magnet strengths.

Magnetic bracelets are not only used for treating arthritis. Searching history vaults revealed that magnetic bracelets have already been utilized for thousands of years. Egyptians and Greeks were the first to report its therapeutic benefits.

In 2000 BC, Chinese texts also revealed that magnets used in acupuncture had yielded positive results. Today, athletes of various sports have expressed their satisfaction after using magnetic bracelets.

Studies have shown that magnetic bracelets are also able to prevent the spread of cancer cells in animals. Lastly, magnetic bracelets have been claimed to successfully treat bacterial infections, stress, and chronic fatigue and magnetic field deficiency syndrome.

To understand the healing process used by arthritis bracelets, you first need to recall your old lessons about magnetic fields. These are produced by various factors like the weather and other natural forces and generated by items like computers, microwave ovens, television sets, and other electronic products.

When exposed to magnetic fields, our bodies experience decreased pH levels and weakened immune systems.

Magnets have both north and south polarities. They come from the two magnetic poles in our world - the North and South Pole. These allow magnetic bracelets to penetrate our skins more easily and have stronger effects.

An arthritis bracelet with the appropriate magnetic strength will create a magnetic field. This magnetic field will then penetrate your skin and reach your muscles and tissues. Any noted inflammation or swelling may be alleviated by the magnetic field.

Some of the things you could enjoy when trying arthritic bracelets include:

Affordability. Compared to other alternative treatments and medications for arthritis, magnetic arthritis bracelets are more affordable. And since they have been acknowledged to be safe to use, there is relatively little harm from trying them out.

Ease of Use or Convenience. It can be tedious having to remember the right time of the day to take your medicine. Fortunately, there's no need for timetables when you're using arthritis bracelets.

The healing process commences the moment you wear an arthritis bracelet, and after that, you need not do anything else.

Improved Circulation. Exposure to magnetic fields allow air and blood to circulate more freely and deliver the necessary nutrients to your organs, blood vessels, muscles, and joints. Better circulation means lesser pain.

Pain. The greatest benefit arthritis bracelets can provide you with is pain relief. This has been supported by data from various studies. There is no need to take a lot or even any painkillers. Pain is eased bit by bit the longer you have your arthritis bracelet on. And with the pain lessened significantly, you'll experience greater freedom of movement.

Lastly, arthritis bracelets also claimed to contain anti-inflammatory properties, potentially making it an aid in solving the root problem of arthritis instead of being simply effective against arthritis symptoms.

CHAPTER 9: CBD HEMP OIL

TREATMENT

There are several proven benefits of Marijuana and its extracts for Arthritis Patients

Although the legal aspects in many countries, funding and other issues inhibit the number of studies on the therapeutic aspects of marijuana, there is still a surprising amounts of information available. The facts so far are clear:

- Marijuana has shown to be an anti-inflammatory
- The potential for cannabis use to help inflammation and muscle spasms have been proven for several illnesses

- Marijuana has been used as a pain treatment for hundreds of years, if not thousands (some records date back to B.C.)

- Studies suggest that marijuana may not only help inflammation, but may lower the actual growth of the disease itself

- Marijuana has historically been used as a pain treatment for rheumatoid arthritis, although its therapeutic potential has not yet been evaluated in any public clinical study.

- THC and CBD, the two main components of marijuana, have been recognized as "key therapeutic constituents that act synergistically together and with other plant constituents."

- THC has shown pain relieving abilities for both nociceptive and neropathic pain.

- CBD has shown the ability to block the progression of rheumatoid arthritis, while both THC and CBD have anti-inflammatory effects.

Cbd hemp oil

CBD, also called Cannabidiol, is just one of 85 different chemical compounds in marijuana plants. CBD Hemp Oil is derived from hemp, or cannabis grown with very little THC (often less than 0.3%). For the sake of this article we will refer to marijuana as cannabis grown for its psychoactive effects, and hemp as cannabis grown for its practical uses as a fiber. Marijuana is marketed for its THC content and hemp is utilized for its CBD content.

THC is the psychoactive or intoxicating compound found in cannabis plants whereas, CBD oil is not psychoactive or intoxicating and has shown strong signs of being an effective treatment for a variety of diseases and mental health disorders.

Cbd hemp oil health benefits

CBD Oil has been shown to have surprisingly positive effects on a variety of diseases. Some of the Cannabidiol health benefits are:

- Nausea treatment
- Lowered anxiety
- Pain relief
- Improved mood
- Lessening withdrawal symptoms
- Seizure reduction
- Stimulating appetite

CBD works by activating the body's serotonin (anti-depressant effect), vanilloid (pain relief), and adenosine (anti-inflammatory effect) receptors. How quickly you start to feel the results from CBD Oil depends on how it was ingested and your weight. Someone small who ingested the oil in spray form will feel the effects much faster than a larger person ingesting CBD in capsule form. CBD Hemp oil has been known to cure 90% of the symptoms of commonly known types of arthritis.

Forms of cbd hemp oil

CBD Hemp Oil can take on many different forms, including liquids, ointments, and sprays, and capsules. Most oils and sprays are used by putting the substance under your tongue.

Ointments are used on and absorbed by the skin, and thirdly capsules are ingested. Those who don't like the taste of sprays or oils can defer to capsules. Capsules are a very convenient way to consume Cannabidiol, however you don't absorb as much CBD from a capsule as you do from an oil or spray put under your tongue.

CBD vape oil is the same as regular CBD Hemp Oil - it's just taken into the body in a different way. You just fill your vape pen with Cannabidiol and presto, you've got yourself a vape with health benefits.

Cbd hemp oil side effects

While not much research has been done yet on the side effects of CBD Oil, whether absorbed, swallowed as a capsule or inhaled through a CBD vape pen, the most commonly side effects reported are digestive issues, such as upset stomach and diarrhea, which are not very common.

CBD Hemp oil and drug Test

Most of you with sensitive jobs may be worried about been accused of doing drugs. Actually, Drug tests are looking for THC, not CBD, and because CBD doesn't produce any kind of high, employers really have no reason to look for it in the first place. So CBD Oil does not show up on a drug test. However, for this reason, make sure you purchase pure CBD oil with 0% THC.

Benefits of Using Pure CBD Oil

No prescription required: Even though they are more potent than regular CBD Oils, most pure CBD Oils do not require a prescription.

0% THC: If you're worried about using a cannabis extract because you don't want to experience marijuana's psychoactive effects or fail a drug test, opt for pure CBD Oil. Containing no THC at all, it's the safest choice.

Fewer side effects: Pure CBD Oils are less likely to cause nausea and fatigue.

Where to Get CBD Hemp Oil

Hemp oil is legal in all 50 states but the production of CBD Hemp Oil is not. Even though both come from marijuana, hemp oil is derived from sterile cannabis seeds, which are legal under the Controlled Substances Act. CBD Oil is derived from the plant's flowers which are not legal in some states. However, this doesn't stop the import of CBD oil made from industrialized hemp grown legally, which is why you're able to buy it legally on the internet.

You can find products containing hemp oil in the beauty section of your local retail store, but to get CBD Oil you'll either need to be in a state where it's legal to produce or purchase an import.

How to identify quality CBD Hemp Oil online

CBD Oil sold online are not as potent as those medically prescribed for serious diseases but they can help with mood disorders, lower anxiety, and lessen pain caused by inflammation.

- Your first clue is usually price. If the price seems too cheap to be true, it probably is.

- Always purchase from a reputable source. A company that is reputable will back their product and will not risk selling misrepresented items.

- Another thing to look for is the way that the product is marketed. If you see CBD Hemp Oil online that claims to cure every ailment under the sun, it's also probably too good to be true.

- The top products are made from organically grown hemp and have a CBD concentration over 20mg.

While the medicinal effects of Cannabidiol are great, keep your expectations of online brands realistic.

Final note

Only a doctor can truly diagnose whether you have Arthritis, and because there are over 100 forms of Arthritis, it is also important to determine which form of Arthritis you have. The different forms of Arthritis have different symptoms as well (above).

It is also important to seek medical treatment as soon as possible, since Arthritis has no known cure, the sooner you seek treatment and begin a regimen of care, and the better your results of managing your Arthritis will be.

Your treatment plan may include things such as a specific course of medicine, plenty of rest, adequate diet, and proper nutrition, losing weight if you are overweight, and in severe cases, surgery may be

Furthermore, regular exercise can play a vital role in the prevention and treatment of all forms of arthritis.

Exercise is essential for reducing pain and retarding joint deterioration and helps to prevent stiffness. But you also need to respect your body's limitations in order for exercise to be beneficial. Exercise helps to keep joints healthy by encouraging the flow of synovial fluid into and out of the cartilage, and strengthens the supporting, protecting structures (muscles, tendons, ligaments) and increases the range of motion, shock absorption, and flexibility of joints.

Exercise is important in both the prevention and treatment of arthritis because unused joints tend to stiffen. Proper instruction is essential, since great harm can be done with what could be a normally easygoing activity. Swimming, water exercise, yoga and tai chi have been found to be slow and careful enough to loosen joints without causing additional discomfort.

Made in the USA
San Bernardino, CA
26 November 2018